Smarter And Wiser Not Harder:

A Guide To Getting The Body And Mind That You Want

By

LINDA A. ROBERTS

Copyright © by Francis K. Pitts 2022. All rights reserved.

TABLE OF CONTENTS

Introduction

Remain grounded and inquisitive.

At the heart of chaos, be the monk who knows how to meditate.

When you witness anything that seems foolish, react to it with kindness.

Which personality type do you aspire to be? This book is meant to assist you in reaching your answer, whatever that may be. Yes, the book is about fitness and health, but it's also about all you can accomplish with greater strength and stamina. Ultimately, the book is about being the finest version of yourself—you, liberated.

Everyone talks about compassion and empathy, but to maintain your best self and keep improving even when things go strange, you must combine these qualities with calmness, curiosity, and a deep sense of mental calm. Because of that combination of attributes, I could comfortably sail through the last few years of extraordinary global change. Together, those attributes form the foundation for leading a decent and contented life. They are just as crucial at difficult times as they are

during seemingly routine days. And you are aware of how hard it is to maintain them continuously. Most of us let them get away without ever recognizing it. Yes, we might occasionally succeed in achieving them, but eventually, the rigors of everyday existence overcome us. We can't allow ourselves to feel at peace because we are too tired.

I've heard folks express a desire to "go back to normal" numerous times during the pandemic, which sounds incorrect each time. That objective is just absurdly modest. I've spent my entire life trying to increase my mental and physical toughness to become better than average and assist others in doing the same. The objective is to raise your baseline, establish it as your new regular, and then raise it again. A crisis is the ideal opportunity to take action. Why would you want to return to the way things used to be?

I also want what I have to be shared with others. To feel replenished rather than exhausted. To lack fear and instead be hazardous. When I say risky, I don't mean that you should take risks like crashing your car or setting your house on fire. You feel free to be who you are, which means you can chase your dreams, be erratic,

and take significant risks. Although it may seem counterintuitive, a significant truth is that being dangerous makes you feel secure and at ease. There is no sense of impending catastrophe when one is dangerous. It takes a lot of energy and grit to be dangerous, which is why so many people believe that a weak

The best they can aspire for is "normal." Luckily, you can also benefit from another fundamental paradox. I like to call it the laziness principle, but the scientific term for it is slope-of-the-curve biology. This book's central concept has the power to change your life. It all comes down to one fundamental yet ground-breaking notion: You can become strong through laziness.
I realize that isn't easy to accept. It's difficult to believe because your body is hiding something from you, a secret. Your body moves more quickly than you do. It takes roughly a third of a second to perceive, process, and respond to inputs before your brain even realizes what it's doing. Your body has sabotaged you before

your logical human brain can apply bravery, willpower, and diligence. It gives you a rush of adrenaline that magnifies even little anxieties. It sends you pain signals to make you believe that simple chores would take a lot

of labor, giving you plenty of excuses not to complete them.

How come your body would sabotage you in that way? Why would Mother Nature design a system that is so cruel? Since everything in the natural world can only be that way. Your body is made to provide you the best chance of surviving, procreating, and continuing the species. Your body, therefore, truly just gives a damn about two things. First, he is not going to die. To avoid dying as much as possible, the second strategy is to be incredibly lazy.

When a predator is going to devour you, your body will not wait for you to make a decision. It will move you away and into safety well before you have time to gather your thoughts and decide how best to respond. Your conscious mind is not in charge of your survival second-by-secondly because it is too slow to react to threats. Your body's autopilot system gives you a tremendous advantage in terms of long-term survival. It is the cause of humanity's continued existence on our planet. But there are a few significant disadvantages.

Section I: Life's Resources

1.

Tap The Power Of Laziness

There are several derogatory names used to characterize lazy people, such as couch potato, bludger, slacker, and so on. Among the seven major sins is sloth. Regardless of your views on moral transgressions, being lazy is viewed negatively in most societies.

But if you take the moral judgment out of it and concentrate on its most fundamental meaning, laziness is just the unwillingness to expend energy. Furthermore, there are benefits to being indolent, many of which have been shown by science.

Why are we lazy?

Although laziness is a typical trait outside of these medical problems, it can be used as a coping method for

depression and anxiety. Even the most driven and diligent individuals occasionally experience laziness. Despite all of these criticisms of laziness, how hard we struggle to attain it is astounding. Why is laziness so ordinary if it's so bad?

Nature has tailored our biological systems to be more indolent. Besides renowned indolent species like pythons, who sleep almost eighteen hours daily, most animals are inactive.

Additionally, there is a direct correlation between the amount of time they spend doing nothing and the time they spend not engaging in activities like hunting, foraging, and reproduction. Compared to relatively unproductive predators, highly efficient predators may appear lazier because they have more leisure time.

The definition of laziness lacks nuance, which is the source of the seeming paradox. Rather than indicating ineffectiveness and lack of productivity, being lazy is frequently the outcome of clever work that frees up time for well-earned rest. Moreover, laziness itself can catalyze intelligent effort.

Progress isn't made by early risers.it`s made by lazy men trying to find easier ways to do something

Despite its seeming paradox, idleness is frequently the opposite of productivity.

Ten advantages of being lazy

Quite the contrary—laziness has its advantages. Being indolent can result in a more contented and productive existence since it can enhance wellness and improve productivity at work. It is long overdue for attitudes regarding laziness to shift.

-Lazy solutions can be smart: Due to laziness, several inventions have come about, including smart speakers, escalators, light switches, and remote controls. The well-known quote by Frank Gilbreth Sr., which is sometimes misattributed to Bill Gates, reads, "I will always choose a lazy person to undertake a tough job because a lazy person will discover an easy way to do it." Although the need is often cited as the mother of creation, idleness also significantly drives innovation.

-One example of active procrastination is slacking off: According to a procrastination study, not all procrastinating actions are detrimental or have unfavorable outcomes. The writers distinguished between two categories of procrastinators: those who put off tasks and those who do not. Those who procrastinate passively do so in the conventional sense. Their inaction paralyzes them, causing them to miss deadlines and fail to finish projects on time.
On the other hand, active procrastinators are a "good" kind of procrastinator. Active procrastinators have excellent time management, coping strategies, and overall performance. They also choose to work under pressure and intentionally choose to put off tasks. It's not too bad for those who are frequently called lazy.

-Those who are lazy concentrate on high-risk endeavors: Those prone to laziness will typically avoid pointless work since they carefully control their energy usage. Alternatively, they do high-leverage jobs with little input and a large output. One way to increase energy is by automating repetitive and time-consuming tasks.

-Time spent on unproductive tasks relieves stress: Studies indicate that putting off tasks and wasting time can be beneficial strategies for managing stress. This is especially valid for teenagers. Young people's mental health requires engagement in activities—or lack thereof—that adults may consider sluggish.

-You are less likely to burn out when you are lazy: Regaining control over one's body and time can be achieved by using boredom and sloth. Lazy people can prevent burnout by allowing their bodies and minds to rest regularly.

-Laziness promotes introspective thinking: The diffuse and focused modes of thought are the two ways our minds might think. To be most creative and productive, we must oscillate constantly between the two phases. Diffuse thought, or mind wandering, is a helpful way for our brains to assimilate information and can occasionally lead to unexpected answers. A better focus on long-term goals is another benefit of letting our minds wander without attending to productive work, according to a study published in Consciousness and Cognition. I have a little downtime now in preparation for tomorrow's more productive period!

-We can benefit mentally from laziness: Maybe the best thing we can do for our mental health is to sit back and relax. Keeping occupied can be a potent defense strategy against unsettling thoughts and emotions. However, when we act in a manic manner, we repress the reality of our emotions and worries and, whether on purpose or not, steer clear of times when our thoughts are free to associate.

-We can replenish our energy reserves by being indolent: Compared to sloth, rest and idleness are not as negatively associated, yet they offer comparable benefits. Numerous studies have demonstrated the health benefits of regular breaks and midday naps, including lowered blood pressure and mental clarity.

-When given enough time to work themselves out, problems can resolve themselves: Sometimes, the best solution to a problem is to put it off, either because it becomes obsolete or because someone who needs the solution more than you will take care of it.

-Being lazy might be a helpful symptom: Our body and mind are sharing vital information when we feel lethargic. Is it that we're hungry or tired? Due to a lack

of drive? Is the work itself tedious or monotonous? One of the best ways to tackle the task more effectively is to acknowledge the sense of sloth. If you lack energy all the time, you might need to look closer at your thoughts and feelings to see what's causing it.

However, don't hold it against yourself if you occasionally feel lethargic. When accepted in a self-compassionate manner, idleness may be both a tool and a key to a deeper understanding of oneself. Despite its many advantages, laziness is an inert state. The environment in which we feel lazy, the task at hand, the amount of time we put it off, and other factors all affect how beneficial or detrimental lethargy can be. Laziness can be used to be more productive and comfortable in the long run, provided it is handled carefully, under control, and without needless shame.

Laziness can result in more creative ideas, wiser choices, and improved mental health.

"I'm a sloth. However, the wheel and bicycle were created by indolent individuals who disliked walking and carrying anything, according to Nobel Peace Prize winner Lech Wałęsa. Be a lazy tactician!

2.

Remove Your Friction

Enhancing oneself is nearly always beneficial. Enhancing minor aspects of your life might have significant outcomes. You can only make so many improvements, though. It's sometimes more effective to remove stuff. Specifically, I'm referring to the removal of friction.

Your net productivity is the balance of the productive and unproductive forces in your life

Thoughts about increasing effort are given a lot of attention and energy, but decreasing friction has many benefits. An automobile will accelerate more quickly if the speed bumps are removed in addition to applying more pressure to the accelerator.

How does one go about living a life with less friction? A simple method is to lessen decision fatigue. It has been demonstrated that decision-making becomes worse the more choices you make. To put it another way, energy is everything. You will have less energy for the vital tasks the more mental and physical energy you expend on the insignificant ones.

Nothing major needs to be involved to remove friction. Little routines build up over time.

- . Set out your clothes the night before
- Plan your meals for the week
- Use auto-pay for your bills
- Delegate unimportant decisions and tasks

- Set a time limit for simple decisions (more time spent picking a restaurant or Netflix show is almost always a waste)
- Once you make a decision, stick with it

Therefore, by all means, continue to enhance the aspects that require improvement. But also give the process of reducing friction some time.

3.

Load Up On Raw Minerals

1. Eating Well to Enhance Focus and Retention
As fast as 268 miles per hour, your brain can process information, as you may have guessed. It needs to be adequately fueled because it is such a crucial organ (that's faster than a Formula 1 race vehicle). These are a few superfoods for brain health, along with their advantages.

2. Energy for Your Mind

The functioning of your brain can be adversely affected by bad dietary choices, just like the rest of your body. Give your brain the proper nourishment to improve concentration and memory:

3. Salmon

Salmon has a relatively high protein content when it comes to brain health. Omega-3 fatty acids, essential for normal brain development and function, are abundant in

fatty fish, such as salmon. These fatty acids have also been shown to reduce the risk of depression, arthritis, and heart disease. The fish are also excellent providers of omega-3 fatty acids: lake trout, mackerel, herring, and tuna.

4. Eggs

There are many beneficial elements in eggs. Regarding brain health, egg yolks are a good source of choline, linked to lowering inflammation and enhancing mental processes, including memory and neuronal transmission. In addition, eggs contain a lot of tryptophan, an amino acid that helps produce serotonin, the chemical known as "happiness." This is a positive side effect that will make you happy.

5. Blueberries

All berries benefit the brain's health, but the blueberry reigns supreme and may have been the first superfood in America. Flavonoids, in particular, are abundant in antioxidants found in blueberries. Increased blood and

oxygen flow to the brain is caused by these antioxidants, which improve concentration. According

to a study, they may even help people with moderate cognitive impairments work better in their minds.

6. Leafy Greens and Cruciferous Vegetables

Leafy greens, which include arugula, kale, and spinach, are high in minerals like folate, beta carotene, and vitamins E and K. Vitamin E shields cells from the harm that free radicals can cause. It has been proposed that these characteristics can stop or slow down the aging population's cognitive deterioration. Memory improvement has been linked to vitamin K. Beta carotene, which aids in delaying the aging process of the brain. Additionally, their antioxidants might shield the brain from harmful free radicals.

7. Nuts

Nuts with unique flavors and textures include macadamias, pistachios, and almonds. Macadamias support healthy brain function, pistachio nut oils maintain fatty acids and reduce inflammation, while almonds aid memory. Still, the walnut wins the best nut,

hands down. Walnuts are richer in DHA, an omega-3 fatty acid that reduces inflammation and have twice the antioxidant content of other nuts, which helps prevent cognitive loss.

8. Coffee

Java fans, rejoice! There are a lot of other advantages to getting a kick start in the morning. By preventing the chemical adenosine, which causes fatigue, from working, caffeine promotes alertness. Researchers at the National Institute on Aging also discovered that people who drank more coffee did better on memory tests. Drink in moderation, as excessive alcohol consumption might have negative consequences.

9. Dark Chocolate

Do you need another reason to eat dark chocolate as a snack? Caffeine, flavonoids, and potent antioxidants can be found in dark chocolate. Flavonoids can improve memory because they increase blood flow to the brain. Caffeine has the potential to enhance short-term cognitive performance.

4.

Supplement Your Brain Power

Who wouldn't want a sharper, more focused brain primed to kill it on trivia night? Thankfully, there are several ways to maintain good brain function. A healthy diet that includes whole grains, fresh produce, and natural proteins is one thing; social gatherings and frequent exercise are two more. However, what if you need a little pick-me-up? Do any supplements that promote brain health? In a nutshell, sure.

Supplements, such as discrete amounts of particular vitamins, minerals, herbs, and probiotics, supply various nutrients. Put differently, they are designed to compensate for any gaps in your diet. It's more challenging than just stocking up if that sounds too good to be true. To optimize the effects and safeguard your health, you must remain aware of everything you put in your body, just like other substances.

For instance, the Food and Drug Administration does not mandate that supplement labels reveal how their products interact with other medications, which could result in unwanted side effects or irritations if medical advice is not obtained promptly. Furthermore, taking too many vitamins might be hazardous in certain situations.

Please speak with your doctor before taking any supplement to determine which nutrients and dosages will support your needs and whether you need them.

Supplement-free mental enhancers

Your doctor will tell you this: supplements are called such for a purpose. Using them as nutritional supplements rather than as a stand-in for a balanced diet is advisable. Thus, before we discuss the top supplements for maintaining brain health, be sure to:

Consume a healthy diet since nutrients from fresh food are far more potent than those found in pills, powders, and chewables. It's frequently tastier and less expensive as well.

Regular exercise is an effective and healthful way to pump blood around your body and brain, distributing nutrients throughout your body. Additionally, it promotes neurogenesis, or the growth of new neurons, which has been linked to improved memory and effects against dementia.

Make sure you get adequate sleep. Research indicates that sleep aids in the removal of toxins that may accumulate in your central nervous system during the day. That explains why you feel refreshed following a restful night's sleep.

Develop your brain by pushing yourself with puzzle games and memory activities. Alternatively, take up a brand-new pastime to exercise your mind every day.

Socialize: Meeting new people is essential to acquiring fresh viewpoints and experiences. It also allows you to impart knowledge to others, which challenges your brain's capacity for concept organization and clear communication.

Three vital nutrients for healthy brain function

What are the ideal foods for the health of your brain, then? A few promote improved creativity, attentiveness, and memory. Others prevent severe mental health disorders from developing. While no single nutrient can accomplish everything, these three can help you become more mentally bright. They may all be purchased as supplements.

Omega-3 fatty acids

Omega-3 fatty acids are an excellent place to start regarding brain vitamins. This is because your body cannot produce this kind of fat alone. And we assure you that you will want to take advantage of their enormous advantages.

Improved brain function, memory, and reaction times are just a few benefits of omega-3 fatty acids. They might also help avoid depression and dementia, as well as lower the chance of Alzheimer's disease. Infants also gain from this. Indeed, omega-3 fatty acids support brain development in the womb and the early years of

life, making them a crucial vitamin for expectant mothers and their unborn children.

Omega-3 fatty fish are great providers of the fatty acids salmon, trout, and herring. However, steer clear of fish high in mercury if you are expecting, nursing, or feeding small children. Among the seafood with the lowest mercury levels are sardines. Not a big fan of fish? There are still a tonne of other omega-3 sources available to you, including flaxseed, soybeans, almonds, and omega-3 pills.

Vitamin D

In addition to its well-known role in maintaining strong bones and preventing osteoporosis, vitamin D has also been connected to normal brain function. Although more studies are needed to comprehend vitamin D's effects on the brain fully, we know much about what happens when we acquire the recommended dosage. In actuality, keeping enough amounts of vitamin D in the body may delay the onset of mental illnesses like dementia, schizophrenia, depression, and Alzheimer's disease. The worst part is that 1 billion or so people worldwide need to receive more of it.

Surprisingly, exposure to sunshine causes your skin to create vitamin D, so taking a five to ten-minute stroll

outside is a great way to get your recommended daily nutrient intake. Various foods, such as egg yolks, cold-water fish (tuna, salmon, and sardines), and morning meal staples, like cereal and milk, also contain vitamin D. Consider taking vitamin D supplements if you have dietary restrictions, have trouble absorbing nutrients, or cannot get outside in the sun.

B12 vitamin

Vitamin B12, like vitamin D, is incredibly beneficial to the brain. Getting adequate vitamin B12 may help you learn new things more efficiently, have more energy, and enhance your memory. Additionally, studies have indicated that it can alleviate depression symptoms and enhance mood. Whole grains, high-fiber cereals, and naturally occurring animal sources like fish, chicken, and dairy may provide you with all the vitamin B12 you require. However, you stand to benefit significantly from supplementing your diet with this powerful brain booster if you're an older adult, vegetarian or vegan or have problems absorbing nutrients.

Section II: Targets and Goals

5.

Pick Your Target

You could wonder where you need to improve and how you'll know when you're headed in the right direction when choosing a target and creating goals for yourself. Additionally, you should ensure that your attempts to better yourself are consistent with your personality and personal values.

Rephrasing your goals as personal growth is one way to make self-improvement goals work. Embracing it can help your personal and professional lives. You must choose a target and create attainable goals that enable you to gain new abilities if you want to grow and improve. This can push you beyond your comfort zone. Setting and achieving personal objectives requires work, discipline, and attention. This is the way to get going.

What are one's objectives?

Your efforts are being directed toward a goal. For example, your objective can be to reach a specific professional benchmark or set a new personal record for how long you run in the morning. You can have personal goals in any aspect of your life.

Furthermore, a personal aim is personal, as the term suggests. The only person you are competing against is yourself. Combining short- and long-term objectives is necessary while setting personal goals.

Assume that although you don't think of yourself as a morning person, you want to start waking up at 5 a.m. It's not feasible to go from getting up ten minutes before your first meeting to adhering to a three-hour morning routine. However, if you get up 30 minutes earlier every month, you'll have a reasonable short-term goal that builds toward your long-term goal. Research indicates that achieving goals is more positively correlated with well-being than the significance of goals. It works better to be realistic about what you can do to maintain motivation.

Being more conscious also increases your chances of succeeding in your endeavors. According to some studies, thoughtful individuals make better, more realistic goals.

You may maintain your mental health for the remainder of your life by making efforts to improve it. And achieving sustainable goals necessitates introspection and inner work. To do Inner Work, one must become more self-aware. The best way to improve yourself is to know who you are.

Take time to acknowledge and feel grateful for the skills you now possess. Instead of attempting to change who you are, you are attempting to support yourself through the various phases of life.

6.

Hack Target: Strength And Cardiovascular Fitness

How does it benefit me?
Aerobic (cardiovascular) exercise:

- Boosts your endurance and vitality
- aids in blood pressure regulation
- enhances the lipid profile of your blood (cholesterol)
- It aids in increasing your caloric expenditure to keep your weight stable.

Cardiovascular exercise has many advantages, but some exercises are appropriate or safe for some people. You should speak with your physician before starting any workout regimen. The contents of this handout should be used in something other than personalized medical advice.

Which type of physical activity will help me get more cardiovascular fitness?

Exercise that works the heart is any action that:
• engages the body's big muscles, particularly the legs.
• has a continuous, rhythmic quality (as opposed to stop-and-start)
• makes your lungs and heart work harder.

"Pure" aerobic exercises include walking, running, jogging, cycling, swimming, aerobics, rowing, stair climbing, hiking, cross-country skiing, and various forms of dancing. Participating in sports like tennis, basketball, squash, and soccer can help increase your cardiovascular fitness. On the other hand, endurance training might enhance these sports performance. Athletes commonly employ three training techniques to enhance their cardiovascular fitness:

- Moderate to sluggish distance training
- Interval training at a moderate to high intensity
- Constantly performing high-intense exercise.

Which kind of cardiovascular workout is the best?

Any workout that you enjoy and will stick with is the best! Choose an exercise that is appropriate for your current level of fitness, health, and personal preferences. Think back to past injuries. Combine weight-supported exercises like cycling and rowing with high-impact ones like step aerobics or running. Your level of aerobic challenge increases with the number of muscles used in the exercise. Cross-country skiers, for instance, have demonstrated the highest aerobic capacity of all sports. They heavily use their arms, legs, and trunk muscles during activity. Among the most significant modifications that occur during cardiovascular exercise

Does the efficiency with which active muscles absorb and use oxygen increase? Most of your training should entail running if you're preparing for a road race, employing the same muscles and movements needed to compete. Swimming or cycling can help reduce the impact on your knees, hips, and feet. However, the best "sport-specific" training for a running event comes from running itself.

For what duration should I work out?

If you're starting, 15 minutes of cardiovascular activity might help you become more stamina. To ensure an increase in aerobic capacity in around 8 to 12 weeks, cardiovascular training necessitates at least 30 minutes three times a week, according to the majority of research. Depending on their fitness level, athletes who use high-intensity continuous training to raise their lactate threshold should work out for 25 to 50 minutes. Low- or high-intensity intervals lasting at least 60 to 90 seconds should be incorporated into interval training to increase aerobic power, with one to two minutes of rest time in between. Collaborate with an experienced fitness specialist to determine the quantity and duration of your training and recovery periods.

On what days of the week should I work out?

Performing aerobic exercises three to five times a week helps enhance your cardiovascular health. There is a higher chance of injury in high-impact activities more than five days a week. Choose two or three exercises that work different muscles and movements if your goal is to work out five or six times a week. This will stop

long-term tension in the muscles and joints. Switch between activities with high and low impact. Exercise is more enjoyable when you have a range of possibilities, significantly as the seasons or circumstances change. Maintaining your current level of aerobic fitness can be achieved with just two days of training each week. Performing high-intensity interval training at most twice a week is recommended. This should only be done once you have a solid foundation of cardiovascular fitness.

7.

Hack Targets: Energy Level And Metabolism

Metabolism is the process by which your body uses the food and liquids it has consumed to produce energy. The link between calories consumed by the body and calories expended by it (i.e., during physical activity) to meet our daily energy needs is known as energy balance. The energy needed for the body to build and repair itself ultimately comes from food.

Your metabolism determines how much energy, expressed in kilojoules (kJ), your body burns at any moment. Reaching and keeping a healthy weight requires finding a balance. When we consistently consume more calories than our body uses for metabolism, most calories are stored as fat. Our body uses most of its energy daily to maintain all its systems in good working order. We have no control over this. But when we exercise, we can force our metabolism to

work in our favor. The body uses more energy (kilojoules) when you are moving.

Like all living things, our bodies are devices for converting energy. According to the energy conservation theory, the chemical energy contained in food is either transformed into thermal energy or stored as energy in fatty tissue.

The rate at which a person's body burns calories to produce energy is known as their metabolism. Age, degree of activity, genetics, and other variables affect how quickly the body breaks down food. Sleep, exercise, and a regular diet help to increase metabolism. The body requires energy from calories to move, breathe, digest food, circulate blood, grow cells, heal wounds, and even think. Several formulas can calculate resting metabolic rate (RMR) or resting energy expenditure (REE), the pace at which the body burns calories to produce this energy. The terms RMR and REE describe how much energy the body expends at rest, such as sitting or sleeping. The rate can differ from person to person. Age, sex, and the activity the person is engaged in are among the variables that influence it.

Although a person's genetic makeup cannot be changed, research indicates that specific tactics can help increase the rate at which the body burns calories.

It is important to remember that even while increasing metabolism might aid in weight loss and calorie burning, it must be used with a balanced diet and frequent exercise.

Ten methods that could aid in boosting metabolism

Eat at regular intervals: Eating at regular intervals helps lower inflammation, enhance circadian rhythms, boost the body's resistance to stress, and regulate gut flora—the mix of bacteria that aid in maintaining a healthy gut.

- Consume breakfast.
- Eat the majority of foods high in energy early in the day.
- Consume two to three meals a day at consistent intervals.
- having fasting periods

Consume adequate calories: Skipping meals can help people lose weight. On the other hand, metabolism may suffer as a result. A similar thing might happen when you eat empty meals. A person's metabolism may slow down if they consume too few calories for their body to store energy.

Increase your protein intake: Cutting calories won't necessarily raise your metabolic rate, but what you eat can. For instance, protein may encourage thermogenesis—the body's process of burning calories—more so than fat or carbs.

Drink green tea: Green tea extract has the potential to accelerate the metabolism of fat. In other ways, it might support healthy weight management. As an illustration:
- You can reduce sugar by drinking green tea instead of sugar-filled drinks and sodas.
- Staying hydrated can be facilitated by consuming green tea throughout the day.
- Green tea's antioxidants may help lower the risk of heart disease, blood pressure, cholesterol, inflammation, and cell damage.

Engage in resistance training: Strength training promotes muscle growth and may marginally raise resting metabolic rates, such as those experienced while sitting or sleeping. The metabolic rate increased slightly when resistance exercise and nutritional changes were combined, but this rise was not statistically significant. Individuals who solely engaged in resistance training experienced decreased fat mass and increased lean mass.

Drink adequate water: The body must be adequately hydrated to perform at its peak. In addition to being essential for a healthy metabolism, water can aid in weight loss.

Reduce stress: Stress can lead to the body producing more cortisol than usual and can also impact hormone levels. One hormone that aids in controlling hunger is cortisol—abnormally elevated cortisol levels in individuals with eating disorders. When under stress, the body releases cortisol. Stress may also have an indirect effect by changing sleep and food habits, which both have the potential to change metabolic rates.

Get enough sleep: Individuals with inferior sleep quality may have slower metabolisms. When people sleep less, their body lowers their metabolic rate to conserve energy, which may result in weight gain.

Get enough vitamins: Make sure you are getting enough vitamins because they are vital for metabolism. Low levels of several B vitamins may affect how quickly the body breaks down fats like cholesterol and triglycerides.

Spice up your meals: Consuming foods high in capsaicin, like chili, can raise your body's metabolic rate, which affects how quickly it burns fat and utilizes energy.

Seek treatment for hypothyroidism since a slowed metabolism can result from low thyroid hormone levels. The synthesis of chemicals that raise body temperature, respiration rate, and oxygen consumption is stimulated by thyroid hormone. This entails using energy at a faster rate. On the other hand, a hypothyroid person's body probably burns energy more slowly. They might have a slower metabolic rate and a greater chance of gaining weight and becoming obese.

Section III: Endless Improvements

8.

Spiritual Strength

Discussions about spirituality are commonplace. Most people see it as a way of life that brings them serenity and a sense of unity with a higher power. It all depends on your level of spiritual strength. However, what is spiritual strength, and how can one develop and fortify one's spirit?

We'll review everything you need about spiritual strength right here. From what it is to the obstacles and ways to overcome them in ways you may not have previously considered. So tune in to learn everything there is to know about spirituality and developing spiritual strength.

What Is Spiritual Strength?

Let's try to understand the fundamentals of spiritual strength before going into any further information. When we discuss spirituality, we often discuss concepts like inner belief and connecting with a higher power. The comprehension and awareness that we are a component of something bigger and more interconnected than ourselves.

Consequently, the strength of your inner convictions is correlated with your spiritual strength. Ideally, People should strive to be as strong spiritually as possible, but that isn't easy. In actuality, strengthening your spirituality frequently requires much commitment and adequate study and practice. Spiritual strength refers to the strength of your inner convictions. Individuals want to ensure they follow their spiritual path to the fullest extent possible. But it also has a unique set of difficulties made worse by the nature of the loud, technologically-driven world we live in today.

Why Should You Direct Your Attention To Your Spiritual Ability?

Your inner strength is just as vital as your physical, mental, emotional, and character strength. It serves as the cornerstone for everything else in your life and a means for you to accomplish a great deal.

Your spiritual essence is the most elusive and challenging aspect of ourselves to focus on since it is unaffected by any bodily aspect, idea, or emotion. But as we will soon show, there are enormous benefits to strengthening your spiritual strength.

Helps To Find A Sense Of Purpose

When you strongly believe in something, you usually have a clearer idea of what you want to accomplish in life. Every action you take is motivated by a purpose, and you always act by your beliefs. This extends beyond religious possibilities to include all forms of self-actualization and life goals.

Gaining a more profound comprehension of your convictions helps you formulate objectives centered on particular principles. Since you are following your intuition and gut feeling, you will undoubtedly become

more conscious of your purpose in life and your desired way of living. You can discover possibilities you were unaware of if you allow your intuition, the voice of your inner spiritual element, to lead you.

As they say, something doesn't necessarily exist just because you haven't seen it before—just like a black swan that can instantly change your reality.

Coping System

Spirituality provides you with a great way to deal with a variety of situations. You can find inner spirituality and a way to deal with any situation, whether happy or sad, trying to let go of past failures, or anything else.
You would understand the sense of knowing someone is always there for you, no matter where you are, if you believe in a higher power. It is beneficial in dealing with different challenges and setbacks in life because it helps you focus on the things that are truly important in life and the fleeting phases or illusions.

Puts An Emphasis On The Good

As you delve deeply into growing your spiritual strength, you will discover that it provides a far more

-positive aspect of life. You discover that you are more appreciative of and understanding of all the beautiful things in life. This guarantees that you feel generally more upbeat, aiding your personal development.

When you realize that everything in the world is in harmony and has a purpose, you start to feel less and less like you need to survive and compete. You realize that nothing can ever threaten you because you are an infinite being. The same is true of everything and everyone around you; they are all just pieces of the puzzle, unique in their own right, just like you are—neither good nor bad.

9.

The Upgrade of the Next Level

First, Become Informed

When you have an objective you would like to accomplish, be it in your career, relationship, or hobby, you should educate yourself on it to decide on the best course of action. On the other hand, you must understand where you are now, where you want to be in the future, and how you plan to get there if you want to take your life to the next level. Therefore, you must examine the first steps and acquire the necessary skills to get to where you want to go. Prioritize lifelong learning and educate yourself through experiences, knowledge, and information.

#2 Transform Thoughts Into Action

Thinking about improving your life to the next level is one thing, but carrying it out is another. It's possible that you were able to advance mentally, but once you

take action and advance physically, your life will catch up. Remember, that doesn't mean you jump into action without giving it any thought. The best course of action is planning your route and then going toward your destination with deliberate steps.

#3 Don't Put Things Off

A bad habit that prevents us from completing tasks, activities, and eventually our goals and dreams is procrastination. If you are prone to procrastinate, you must make up for lost time instead of tackling previously easily accomplished tasks. You must get over your procrastination and get things done immediately if you want to improve any aspect of your life. Nothing should be put off until tomorrow because it never comes. This moment, this now is all that ever really matters. Nothing more.

#4 Embrace Your Fears

Fears are the most significant obstacle keeping you from moving to the next level. On a personal level, many people are hesitant to share their feelings with friends, but it only keeps you from developing your

friendship. As Dr. Seuss has already stated, "Those who care don't matter, and those who matter don't care." The same is true in your career, so don't fear your friend's response or rejection. Don't give up because you're worried about being rejected or failing. To succeed and advance in life, you must bravely face your fear. Only then can you overcome your fear.

#5 Get Accustomed to Being Uncomfy

Although we can enjoy how comfy our current reality is, it prevents us from taking risks and being courageous. You will need to push yourself harder than ever, forgo some sleep, skip some enjoyable times, and devote more time to studying to take your life to the next level. It's not always easy, but to advance and be open to new concepts, you must learn to be uncomfortable because suffering is a necessary part of growth. Remember that the brief discomfort will pass, and you will soon arrive at your objective when you experience an entirely new degree of ease.

#6 Seek Out a Guide

Finding a mentor who can impart their knowledge to you is one of the quickest methods to take your life to the next level. Locate an expert in the area you wish to improve, and take as much advice as possible from them. While it's understandable that you want to have your own experiences and forge your path, wouldn't it be fantastic to learn from a mentor and reduce the length of your learning curve by half? Remember that mentors are there to assist you in taking your life to the next level, so make sure you use this valuable resource.

#7 Concentration

We must know what it looks like to elevate our lives to the next level. It is crucial to have a clear goal in our minds and pursue it with all of our might—heart, mind, soul, and strength. Moving on to the next level will be possible if you prioritize improving your life and eliminate any outside distractions.

#8 Maintain Consistency

We know what we need to do to take our lives to the next level, but we must continually demonstrate excellent behaviors to get there. True, unforeseen events might derail us from our goals, but the more diligent you are in completing your tasks, the quicker and more successfully you will advance to the next level of accomplishment. Just consider this: where would you be today if you had acted consistently in the past? Continue to follow your plan and make it even better.

#9 Examine Your Way of Life

Science has repeatedly demonstrated that nutrition and exercise are essential for mental and physical well-being. Therefore, we must pay attention to this information to take our lives to the next level. Remember that you can only advance if you have the energy to do it, so prioritize your mental, emotional, and physical well-being. Engage in daily physical activity, maintain a nutritious diet, abstain from alcohol, sip copious amounts of water, peruse motivational literature, view inspiring films, and tune into uplifting

-podcasts. Verify that your lifestyle choices align with your desire to improve your lot in life.

#10 Foster an Upbeat Environment

You'll get where you're going with positivity and optimism. Maintaining a constructive and healthy viewpoint will help you stay strong and motivated by establishing an environment favorable to positivity, optimism, and success. In addition to motivating you and lowering your stress level, having a positive outlook will help you balance where you are now and where you want to be in the future.

There will always come a moment, whatever you do in life, when you need to step it up. Eventually, you want to advance, even if everything is going well. Regardless of who you are, each stage of life calls for a different you, so push yourself to achieve your personal and professional goals.

NEVER SETTLE FOR LESS!

10.

You Do You

Being who you are is positive because attempting to be someone else usually doesn't work out.

But how do you do it?

It would help if you first recognized the things you have unlearned about yourself. This process might be depressing since it brings to mind past choices you made when you could have been who you were, but instead, you decided to be someone else.

Why not start by following your inner compass and doing nothing else, as striving to be someone else is usually futile? What would a day in your life look like if you committed to it entirely?
Some ideologies contend that you are essentially evil and must constantly fight against your true nature,

-making it impossible to make moral decisions on your own. You need help of any type to succeed.

But what if you were a good person at heart? Although you have made mistakes more than most, this does not indicate that you will always make poor choices. Are you not able to follow your convictions with integrity? You can be a good person, aren't you?

Everybody knows at least one resentful, unfavorable person. According to my theory, most resentful people are not being authentic. I hypothesize that they made a poor decision somewhere down the line that they have always regretted, and they vent their displeasure on other people. You know how one guy can tell you you're foolish every time you don't know how to do something? You have to be able to look past that guy and be yourself.

Remorse is the second-last thing you want, but bitterness is the final thing you want. It is up to you to take proactive measures to prevent regret. Progress is preferable to stagnation. Furthermore, I believe that

showing someone you care about them is necessary— just thinking kind thoughts about them is ineffective.

It's dangerous to be who you are. Whose fault would it be if something went wrong? (This is another reason it could be simpler to delegate decision-making to others;

if something doesn't work out, you can always point the finger at them.)

But you know you can be a nice person in the long term. You are confident in your ability to accept the danger. You can find the path to follow the life and career you've always wanted, even if some individuals don't understand.

And today, you can be who you are, yourself.

Conclusion

We've been able to go over a few essential hacks, and shown how beating your innate lazy tendencies may be achieved by being "smarter and wiser, not harder." However, how can you tell if you're improving by evaluating your performance on predetermined goals?

For instance, what is your resting heart rate in terms of cardio? Has your one-rep maximum improved in terms of strength? Your feelings alone will tell you whether or not you have more energy. How do you do on memory and reaction speed tests for your brain? Lastly, use a home monitor to measure your heart rate variability about stress.

Finally, remember to customize your hacks and see what works best for you. Make sure you never stop getting better. Your new baselines should not satisfy you; there is always space for improvement.